# The Plant-Based Diet Mastery

*Top Health And Delicious Plant-Based Diet Recipes To Reset & Fortify Your Body With A Simple Meal Plan*

**Amy Instant**

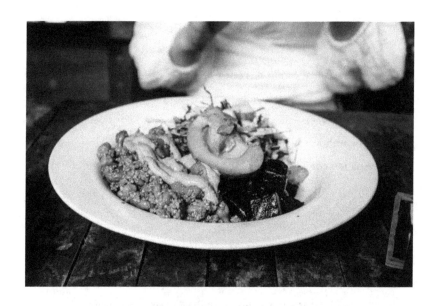

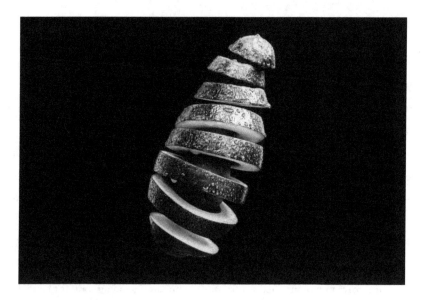

# Table of Contents

INTRODUCTION..................................................................... 8

WHY PLANT-BASED DIET? ...........................................................9

TYPES OF PLANT-BASED DIET .....................................................9

BENEFITS OF A PLANT-BASED DIET................................................10

PLANT -BASED DIET BLUE PRINT..................................................12

HEALTH BENEFITS OF THE PLANT-BASED DIET ..............................18

METABOLIC SYNDROME ............................................................19

HIGH BLOOD PRESSURE............................................................20

CARDIOVASCULAR DISEASE .......................................................21

CHAPTER 1.    BREAKFASTS ................................................... 26

1.    GREEN CROQUETTES...........................................................26

2.    CIGAR BOREK.................................................................28

3.    FLAKED CLUSTERS.............................................................30

4.    MARINARA SAUCE.............................................................32

5.    ENCHILADA SAUCE............................................................34

6.    MEXICAN SALSA ..............................................................36

7.    APPLE SAUCE.................................................................38

8.    VEGAN MAYO..................................................................40

9.    CHICKPEA VEGGIE OMELETS...................................................42

10.    MAPLE CINNAMON FRENCH TOAST .............................................45

11.    SAVORY SWEET POTATO OVEN HASH ..........................................48

12.   LEMON POPPY SEED PANCAKES ...................................................................50

**CHAPTER 2.   : SALADS, SOUPS, AND SIDES ........................................... 54**

13.   ZUCCHINI SOUP ........................................................................................54

14.   CREAMY CELERY SOUP ...........................................................................56

15.   AVOCADO CUCUMBER SOUP ...................................................................58

16.   CREAMY GARLIC ONION SOUP ...............................................................60

17.   AVOCADO BROCCOLI SOUP .....................................................................62

**CHAPTER 3.   : ENTRÉES ......................................................................... 64**

18.   SUPER TASTY VEGETARIAN CHILI ............................................................64

19.   CREAMY SWEET POTATO & COCONUT CURRY ............................................66

20.   COMFORTING CHICKPEA TAGINE ............................................................69

21.   BROWN BASMATI RICE PILAF ..................................................................72

22.   MEXICAN RICE .......................................................................................74

23.   ARTICHOKE & EGGPLANT RICE ...............................................................76

24.   BLACK BEANS AND RICE .........................................................................79

**CHAPTER 4.   : SMOOTHIES AND BEVERAGES ................................... 82**

25.   SPICED STRAWBERRY SMOOTHIE .............................................................82

26.   BANANA BREAD SHAKE WITH WALNUT MILK ............................................84

27.   DOUBLE CHOCOLATE HAZELNUT ESPRESSO SHAKE ...................................85

28.   STRAWBERRY, BANANA AND COCONUT SHAKE .........................................87

29.   TROPICAL VIBES GREEN SMOOTHIE .........................................................88

**CHAPTER 5.    : SNACKS AND DESSERTS .............................................. 90**

30.   VEGAN FUDGE REVEL BARS............................................90

31.   NORI SNACK ROLLS..........................................................92

32.   RISOTTO BITES .................................................................94

33.   TAMARI TOASTED ALMONDS..........................................96

34.   KALE CHIPS.......................................................................98

35.   SAVORY SEED CRACKERS .............................................100

36.   MUSHROOM BITES .........................................................102

**CHAPTER 6.    : SAUCES, DRESSINGS, AND DIPS .............................. 104**

37.   RASPBERRY SAUCE.........................................................104

38.   BABA GANOUSH..............................................................106

39.   BASIL PESTO ...................................................................108

40.   POPPY SEED DRESSING .................................................110

41.   CRANBERRY DRESSING .................................................112

**CONCLUSION .................................................................................. 114**

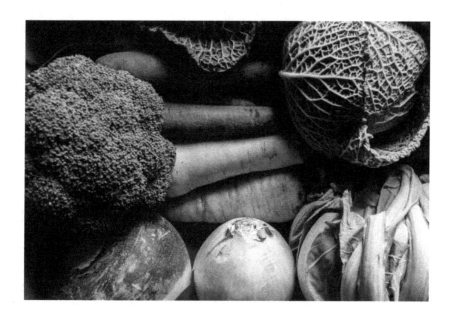

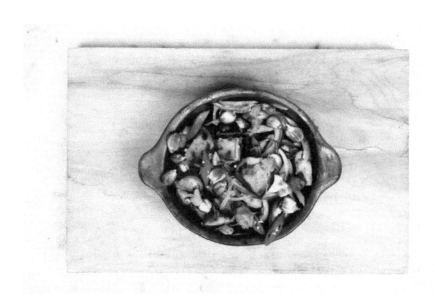

# Introduction

Plant-based diet can vary from one person to another. However, the foundational idea is that we try to avoid processed food as much as possible and choose to use what we receive from the beautiful planet that we live in. By that, I mean the incredible ingredients derived from the earth. In essence, plant-based diet comes with a few benefits. Plant-based diet avoids using processed foods as much as possible. There are no animal products in the diet. The categories that are majorly included are vegetables, fruits, seeds and nuts, legumes, whole grains, and herbs and spices. The diet tries to limit the use of sugar, wheat-flour, and oil as much as possible. It focuses on the quality of food, mostly utilizing locally or farm-produced organic foods An important thing to remember here is that there are minimally processed foods included in the plant-based diet, such as non-dairy milk, tofu, and whole-wheat paste, to name a few. Overall, we aim to keep processed foods where they belong: on supermarket shelves, not in our refrigerators. When people look at the list of foods that come in a plant-based diet, they are often focused on how little we have to work on. However, that is probably due to the fact that many of the meat options have suddenly been removed. It feels as though a major part of the diet has been excluded due to it. How can life be fun without a nice steak? What can we do without chicken wings? Is there anything that can be done without a delicious fish? In reality, there are numerous ingredients that you can work with. Additionally, the fun is not just in the ingredients but how we prepare them. The growing demand has seen a rise in people trying out new recipes and mashing up ingredients in interesting ways. Have you heard of smoothies that contain cayenne pepper? Sounds pretty exciting, doesn't it? We are going to look at such wonderful and delicious recipes along with so many more dishes that use wholesome and natural ingredients. Some people are doing it; some people are talking about it, but there is still a lot of confusion about what a whole plant-based diet actually entails. Since we split food into their macronutrients: sugars, proteins, and fats, most of us are uncertain about nutrition. What if we were able to put these macronutrients back together again in order to free your mind from confusion and stress? The secret here is simplicity.

Plant Based Diet
A plant-based diet is a diet that comprises lots of products from plants, and very little or no amounts of animal products and processed foods.

## Why plant-based diet?

Research suggests that those eating a plant-based diet tend to have a lower Body Mass Index (BMI) and therefore are slimmer, healthier and more energetic. Additionally, this means they tend to have lower rates of diabetes, heart disease and stroke than those who eat diets based around meat, especially processed meats.

This may be because plant-based foods such as fresh vegetables, fruits and nuts tend to be higher in complex carbs and fiber so keep you feeling fuller for longer. When you're full, you're far less likely to reach for unhealthy foods that won't nourish your body or mind.

They're also high in antioxidant, vitamins and minerals which are in a natural state and so more readily absorbed by the body.

Additionally, a plant-based diet has been shown to help reduce cholesterol, reduce high blood pressure and even certain types of cancer.

## Types of Plant-Based Diet

Vegan: Diet includes vegetables, seeds, nuts, legumes, grains, and fruit and excludes all animal products (i.e. no animal flesh, dairy, or eggs). There are variations within the vegan diet as well such as the fruitarian diet made up mainly of fruits and sometimes nuts and seeds and the raw vegan diet where food is not cooked.

Vegetarian: Diet includes vegetables, fruit, nuts, legumes, grains, and seeds and excludes meat but may include eggs or dairy. The Ovo-lacto vegetarian diet incorporates dairy and eggs while the Ovo-vegetarian diet incorporates eggs and excludes dairy and the lacto vegetarian diet incorporates dairy but excludes eggs.

Semi-vegetarianism: Diet is mostly vegetarian but also incorporates some meat and animal products. The macrobiotic diet is a type of semi-vegetarian diet that emphasizes vegetables, beans, whole grains, naturally processed foods, and may include some seafood, meat, or poultry. The pescatarian diet includes plant foods, eggs, dairy, and seafood but no other types of animal flesh. People who subscribe to a semi-vegetarian diet sometimes describe themselves as flexitarians as well.

Difference between plant-based diet and vegan, vegetarian diet

A plant-based diet is all about easy healthy plant food option that includes fruits, vegetables, lentils, beans, and more. Other than the hardcore plant diet options, it allows the intake of low-fat dairy products that includes low-fat milk, low-fat cottage, mozzarella and cheddar cheese as well. Having a plant-based diet doesn't require that you avoid all the animal-based products.

A vegan diet states that one should eat all the vegetables and avoid any meat products. It is simply that a person prefers eating vegetables and fruits instead of meat and other fats. Vegan culture involves not using any other animal products not in food nor any daily use.

A vegetarian diet is about focusing on plant foods but also eating animal products such as honey and milk. The main difference with veganism is that vegans avoid any form of animal products while vegetarians do not eat meat but they eat animal products like honey and milk.

## Benefits of a Plant-Based Diet

• Environmentally friendly: Plant-based diet is all environmentally friendly. When masses are following the plant-based diet that means there will be more plants and no more packing food. No processed or packaged food means there won't be any disposal or trash out there. On the other hand, more plants will provide more oxygen for people and give them nutrients through food. It is an overall a good package for the ultimate healthy and happy society.

•      Better organ health: Plant-based diet is good for not only a specific organ like liver, heart or kidneys, but it helps your overall body to have a perfect mechanism. It gives proper attention to all the organs and make it possible for a person to have the best of health in any manner. Other than organs, the diet helps to increase muscular strength, make bones stronger, hair longer and many more. It is all about how you are managing the diet and you will be able to get the best results within a few days of starting with it.

•      Benefits beyond health: The benefits of plant-based diet are not limited to the health and fitness only. It is a complete package of ultimate benefits that prolong in society and help each aspect of the society to grow better. Since the diet is all about plants, it means one needs to have fresh vegetables and fruits available in surroundings. Moreover, it enhances the consumption and utilization of all the products and bi-products. Here are some of the value-added benefits of the plant-based diet that is commendable:

•      Lowers Blood Pressure: One of the reasons why plant-based foods contribute to low blood pressure is that they tend to have high amount of potassium, which in turn helps you manage your blood pressure (Physicians Committee for Responsible Medicine, n.d.). Additionally, potassium has also been known to reduce anxiety and stress. Now, guess what meat has little of? That's right. Potassium. Some foods that have a high amount of potassium are fruits, whole grains, nuts, and legumes.

•      Prevents Chronic Diseases: Obesity? Cancer? Diabetes? These are illnesses that you can avoid or minimize the risk of with a plant-based diet. People who are already suffering from chronic diseases are asked to live on plant-based food because they help improve lifespans (Nordqvist, 2012).

•      Lowers Blood Sugar Levels: One thing that plant-based diets are rich in is fiber. When you consume fiber, your body reduces the amount of sugar it absorbs into the bloodstream. Additionally, fiber does not make you feel hungry really fast. When you do not feel full, you end up consuming more food than necessary. Plant-based foods help prevent such a situation from arising.

• Ideal for Weight Loss: When you are consuming a plant-based diet, you are cutting down on excess fats and maintaining a healthy level of weight. You don't even have to worry about calorie restrictions! Weight loss is possible with a plant-based diet simply because of the fiber we mentioned previously. It helps you manage your hunger, and you also receive the necessary amount of minerals, proteins, and vitamins from your green meal.

• Saves Time and Money: Plant-based foods are not as difficult to prepare as meat-based foods. In fact, you will take less time to prepare an organic meal. When you really need, you can easily put together some healthy ingredients and make a quick salad. Furthermore, you spend less money by preparing food using plant-based ingredients. When you source local and organic products, you end up shelling out less cash for the items that you would like to buy.

• Lowers Cholesterol Level: This might sound like a myth, but plants contain no cholesterol. Even if you pick out coconut and cocoa plants, they do not contain any cholesterol. Hence, when you are at risk of having a high level of cholesterol, a plant-based diet will help you bring it back down to a much healthier level.

## Plant -Based Diet Blue Print

Foods to Eat
Vegetables: tomatoes, cauliflower, spinach, carrots, kale, asparagus, peppers, and broccoli.
Whole Grains: rolled oats, quinoa, pastas made with brown rice, barley, faro, and brown rice, wild rice, amaranth, buckwheat, spelt, kamut, and couscous.
Legumes: chickpeas, peanuts, black beans, peas, and lentils.
Fruits: citrus fruits, bananas, apples, pineapples, berries, and pears.
Starchy Vegetables: sweet potatoes, squash, regular potatoes.
Healthy Fats: avocados, unsweetened coconut, olive oils, and coconut oils.
Seeds: Nut Butters, and Nuts: Macadamia nuts, sunflower seeds, pumpkin seeds, almond butter, cashews, almonds, and tahini.

Plant-Based Milks: almond milk, coconut milk, cashew milk. For this category, it might be tempting to get the sweetened varieties to help you get accustomed to the taste. Initially, that is okay, however, for the long-term, the sweeteners in these milks are not great for your overall health. Perhaps eventually, you can experiment with making some great nut-milk at home, where you can control how much it's sweetened.

Spices and Seasonings: rosemary, turmeric (this spice in particular is great for reducing internal inflammation), curry, sea salt, basil, black pepper.

Drinks: unsweetened coffees and teas, fresh fruit and vegetable juices or smoothies, plain water, sparkling water. There are some great new brands of flavored and sparkling waters available that are sugar-free and help abstain from pop and sweetened juice. No matter what diet you choose, drinking loads of water is great for your body. Additionally, if you really want to boost your immunity and also help your body detox naturally, try adding some berries, sliced orange/lemon/cucumber, mint or lavender to your water. They each make for a tasty flavored water combination either altogether or individually as well.

Condiments: mustard, vegan mayonnaise, soy sauce, tamari, vinegar (apple cider vinegar is wonderful), lemon juice, salsa, and nutritional yeasts.

Plant-based Proteins: tempeh and tofu. A little later, we will provide fabulous recipes for these meatless, yet protein packed, plant-based options.

Foods to Avoid

Animal Foods

Yes, no duh! Being plant-based means that you should avoid animal foods as much as possible. Whether you are doing this for health purposes or for the love of animals, just be sure you try to avoid animal products as much as possible. Some of the more popular options include

Meat: Organs, Veal, Pork, Lamb, and Beef, etc.

Poultry: Duck, Goose, Turkey, Chicken, etc.

Eggs: Any Type of Egg

Dairy: Ice Cream, Butter, Cheese, Yogurt, etc.

Seafood and Fish: All Fish, Lobster, Crab, Mussels, Shrimp, etc.

Bee Products: Honey, Royal Jelly, etc.

Animal Derived Ingredients & Additives: This is where it can get a bit tricky when it comes to living a plant-based diet. One moment you are enjoying one of your favorite snacks, the next you are reading the label and realizing it has an ingredient that has been derived from an animal. Of course, we all make mistakes, but by being educated, you can avoid this mistake in the first place!

Tips to Get Started

As a newbie to plant-based diets, you should understand that this is not something you can just jump into. Your body needs time to adapt to the new style of eating. As you take this important step in your life, here are a few pointers to help you get started.

Find Your Motivation

Before making any changes to your diet, it is essential to take a step back and determine the reasons why you need to make this step. Why do you want to try a plant-based diet? Maybe you are suffering from a disease and this is the best strategy for you to reduce the effects of the disease. Alternatively, it could be that you are looking for a way of improving your health as a means to your overall happiness. Good health means a good heart. It doesn't matter what reasons you have for taking this path. What you need to do is write down your motivation and remind yourself of it every time you wake up.

Start Slow

This is the second most important consideration you should bear in mind. You need to initiate your transition slowly. Select a few foods that are plant-based and begin rotating them for about a week. A good tip here is to select foods that you often enjoy. They can range from lentil stew, oatmeal, jacket potatoes, beans, or veggie stir-fry. Human beings are creatures of habit. Therefore, make a list of the most common plant-based foods that interest you. This should be your starting point as you help your body make a smooth transition.

Cut Down on Processed Foods and Meat

A slow transition guarantees that your body adapts well to the change in diet. In line with this, you shouldn't just avoid processed foods and meat from the get-go. This should be done gradually. Begin by cutting down on your meat intake. Increase the portions of veggies on your plate while reducing the meat portions. After some time, get rid of them entirely as you will have gained the perception that you can do without them. Later on, work on your recipes. If you were a huge fan of beef chili, you can swap the meat with portobello mushrooms. The idea is to continue eating your favorite meals, but as a plant-based version of what you used to have.

Try a Plant-Based Breakfast

After making a few attempts here and there, your next step should be to grab a plant-based meal every day. It would be a good idea for you to start your morning with a vegetarian breakfast. Maybe you are worried that you don't know where to start. There are several plant-based recipes for breakfast, lunch, and dinner that will be provided in this guide. They should help you get started on adopting a plant-based lifestyle.

Surround Yourself with Wholesome Foods

If you are going to adopt a healthy lifestyle, then it is important that you surround yourself with healthy foods. In this case, no other forms of food will be okay; you should only have plant-based foods. Walk around your kitchen as you try and evaluate whether the foods around you are helpful to your goal. If not, don't hesitate to throw them away or donate them. Just because you bought them doesn't imply that you will be wasting food if you choose not to eat them.

Watch Your Protein Portions

The Dietary Reference Intake recommends that the average amount of protein that the body needs is about 0.8 grams per kilogram of body weight. This implies that the typical, sedentary man will require about 56 grams of daily protein intake, whereas a woman will require about 46 grams (Gunnars, 2018). This shows that we only need a fraction of our protein intake to supplement the body with what it needs. Unfortunately, most dieters over-consume proteins with the idea that the body requires the nutrients. What we forget is that too much of something can be toxic and dangerous.

Whether the body needs it or not, watching our portions is vital. While striving to live on a plant-based diet, you should be careful of the amounts of protein you consume. Excessive intake will undeniably lead to negative health effects. What you need to do is make sure that your plant foods have enough calories to provide your body with the energy it needs for metabolism and other purposes.

Educate Yourself

In addition to focusing on food, you should also invest your time and money in educating yourself, just like you are doing by reading this book. It is unfortunate that digital media and advertising has polluted our minds. We are blinded from realizing that plant-based foods are the best foods for our bodies and the planet we live on. Educating yourself is the surest way to get the answers to lifestyle-related questions. You should recognize that, by taking the time to learn, you will be motivated to focus on your goal since you know what you are after.

Find Like-Minded People

Relating to like-minded individuals will be helpful in good and bad times. These are people who are also looking to benefit from eating plant-based foods. Therefore, by relating to them, you can share success stories as well as help each other out in times of need. With the advent of the Internet, it should not be difficult for you to find other people who are vegetarians. Browse through social media pages and join their groups. Here, you will find significant information about your new diet plan. For instance, some people will be eager to share tasty, plant-based recipes with you.

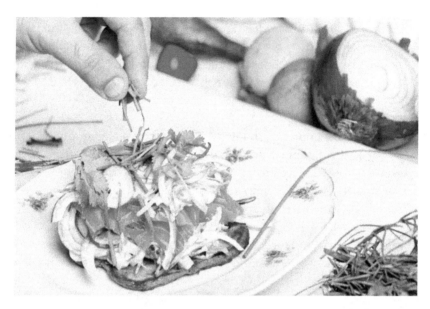

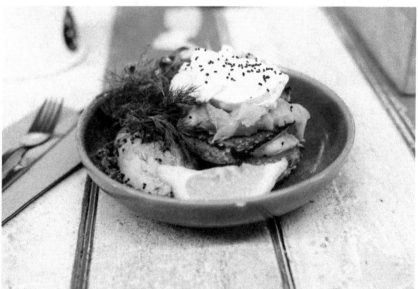

# Health Benefits Of The Plant-based Diet

The primary objective of a healthy, plant-based diet is to minimize the consumption of animal foods, eggs, dairy products, oils, and processed foods while maximizing the consumption of plant foods that are full of needed nutrients. The diet encourages the inclusion of fruits, raw and cooked vegetables, peas, beans, soybeans, lentils, nuts, and seeds. The diet is generally low in fat while being high on the satiety scale, which means the food you eat will fill you up and keep you fuller for longer with fewer calories.

Plants are good for us because they are healthy. Vegetables and fruits are loaded with fiber, antioxidants, minerals, and vitamins. Most people do not regularly consume enough fiber, especially those whose diet is high in processed foods. But besides being full of vitamins and fiber, eating a plant-based diet has other health benefits that will keep you living healthier for longer.

Obesity

Obesity is a medical condition where a person is carrying around more weight than is healthy for them to carry on their bodies. Many people could stand to lose a few pounds, but an obese person has a higher body mass index (BMI) than most people. You will divide your weight in kilograms by your height in meters squared to find your body mass index. There are numerous online calculators that will determine your BMI for you. Generally, anything over twenty-five is considered overweight. If the BMI number is thirty or more, then the person is considered to be obese. Obesity can definitely increase your overall risk of developing many conditions, including high blood pressure, cardiovascular disease, and Type 2 Diabetes.

People become obese for many reasons. The number one cause of obesity is simply consuming too many calories. When you eat more calories than your body needs you to eat to provide energy for your body, then the excess food is stored as fat, and you become obese. Certain types of food are more likely to cause you to be obese, such as foods that are high in sugar and fat. These foods are high in sugar, which is very easy for the body to turn into glucose, or blood sugar, in your body.

When you eat food, your body begins breaking the food down into usable molecules as soon as you begin chewing. When the food reaches your stomach, it encounters various stomach acids that continue to break the food down into tiny particles. After that, the food particles pass into your intestines, where they are either absorbed as usable nutrients or eliminated as waste products. The food particles that are absorbed then move into your bloodstream as glucose, the blood sugar. This glucose is the fuel that the cells need in order to complete their processes and restore themselves. While your stomach was digesting the food, your pancreas was making insulin, which is the hormone the body needs in order to move the glucose into the cells. When the insulin has moved all of the glucose into the cells that the cells will accept, any leftover glucose will be stored as fat in your body. This is a normal function of the body, and it is leftover from the time when food sources were sometimes scarce and the body might not know when it would receive its next meal, so it developed the habit of storing a bit of food for the lean times. When you continuously eat more food, more calories than you need to consume then your body will store more leftover glucose as fat, and you will eventually become obese.

People who follow a plant-based diet weigh less than their meat-eating counterparts and are actually able to eat a larger amount of food. Three ounces of beef weighs in at 213 calories, while three ounces of carrots only has ninety calories. Three ounces of bell pepper gives you seventy-five calories, three ounces of celery is forty-five calories, and three ounces of cucumber brings in thirty calories. Add to this the fact that vegetables are high in fiber, which passes right through the body as a waste product, and it is easy to see how weight can be controlled by following a plant-based diet.

## Metabolic Syndrome

Constantly overeating and being obese will eventually lead to metabolic syndrome. As you eat food, your body makes insulin in order to be able to move the product of the food being consumed, the glucose in your blood, into your cells. The insulin opens the doors of the cells to allow glucose to enter. When food is consumed continuously, or too much food is consumed, insulin is constantly being produced in order to deal with the steady stream of food flowing through the body. Eventually, the cells become full, and they stop responding to the prompt of the insulin. They will accept no more glucose from the blood. So the body has no choice but to store the glucose as fat in the body. This is known as insulin resistance and is one of the major factors in developing metabolic syndrome, which is characterized by having a large waist, from the fat stored underneath the skin, and will eventually lead to the development of life-threatening diseases.

The fiber-rich foods, which include vegetables, nuts, and seeds that are consumed on the plant-based diet, will help to guard against the development of the metabolic syndrome. Following the plant-based diet will lead to a lower weight which in turn will lead to lowered levels of fat and blood sugar. The followers of the plant-based diet will also have less digestive issues, which is another cause of metabolic syndrome.

## High Blood Pressure

In monitoring your overall health, your blood pressure is an important number to know and try to control. There are two individual numbers that are used to measure your blood pressure. The first number, the number on top, is the systolic pressure. The second number, the number on the bottom, is the diastolic pressure. The systolic pressure is the measure of the amount of force, or pressure, which the walls of your arteries undergo when your heart muscle contracts to force the blood to move from the heart and out to the body. The diastolic number measures the amount of pressure that the moving blood puts on your arteries when your heart is resting. So if your heart muscle is working harder to force blood out to the arteries, then your blood pressure reading will be higher than is considered healthy.

High blood pressure is caused by the strain your heart produces, trying to move your oxygenated blood out to all of the cells in your body through the miles and miles of arteries and veins. As people gain weight, their bodies will produce more lengths of arteries and veins so that it is able to supply blood, oxygen, and other nutrients to all parts of your body. If your body did not do these things, then those extra parts of you, like the excess belly fat, would eventually die from starvation. But the body intends for you to keep all of your parts healthy, so it works harder to keep all of you well fed.

When the systolic reading is over 120 and the diastolic reading is over 80, a person is considered to be on their way to developing high blood pressure. Sometimes a reading will be higher if the person is stressed, sick, or has just drunk a hot beverage or smoked a cigarette. But when the reading is constantly higher, then high blood pressure is a real threat. Continuous high blood pressure can lead to kidney disease, strokes, heart problems, and loss of vision. Managing your intake of healthy foods in your daily diet is one of the best ways to naturally lower your high blood pressure. A balanced diet of healthy foods like vegetables, fruits, and whole grains is proven to lower overall body weight and, along with it, high blood pressure. Remember, if the heart does not need to pump blood through all those extra miles of arteries, it won't need to work as hard. And the plant-based diet will provide healthy alternatives to animal fat in the form of omega oil, nuts, and seeds. And foods that are higher in potassium, like bananas, mushrooms, beans, and tomatoes, are known to help lower high blood pressure.

## Cardiovascular Disease

Cardiovascular disease refers to any illness or disease that happens in any part of the cardiovascular system, which is your lungs, arteries, veins, and heart. Most of the issues that involve the cardiovascular disease begin with high blood pressure and a condition known as atherosclerosis. This is a disease of the arteries in the body that is caused by deposits of fatty material known as plaque build-up on the inner walls of the arteries. Plaque buildup is a collection of excess bits of waste products, fat cells, and calcium deposits that collect along the inside walls of your arteries in spots that have become thinned from the force of high blood pressure. Plaque buildup is another thing that will cause the heart to pump faster and harder as it tries to push blood flow past these blockages.

An accumulation of plaque will slow and eventually block the flow of healthy blood through your body, which makes it more difficult for nutrients and oxygen to get to all parts of your body. Another concern involved with plaque buildup is that these formations can eventually break loose and allow little bits of debris to float through your bloodstream. If one of these bits of debris reaches the major arteries n your neck, the blockage could cause you to have a stroke. If one of these blockages reaches the arteries in your heart, then you could suffer a heart attack.

Blood cholesterol is another factor that will lead to good or bad cardiovascular health and is directly affected by your diet. Cholesterol is a wax type of substance that is produced by your liver that helps your body to produce hormones and build membranes for your cells. Your body will naturally produce the amount of cholesterol that it needs, so there is no need to consume excess amounts of cholesterol for the health of your body. When your cholesterol is measured, the doctor is looking at three separate numbers. The first number is your total cholesterol level, which measures the total level of cholesterol in your blood. The second number is the high-density lipoprotein (HDL) level, which is the measurement of the good cholesterol in your blood. The third number is the low-density lipoprotein (LDL) level, which measures the bad cholesterol in your blood. The LDL level is the amount of the bad type of fat that you have floating around in your blood, the type of fat that causes plaque in your arteries.

The benefit of the plant-based diet is that plants are naturally low in fat and contain very small amounts of saturated fat, no dietary cholesterol, and abundant amounts of natural fiber. Saturated fats and cholesterol, which are found in eggs, cheese, and meats, are major contributors to the accumulation of plaque deposits in the arteries, which will eventually lead to some form of cardiovascular disease. The high levels of potassium in plants will help to lower high blood pressure. The high fiber levels in plants will help to lower high blood cholesterol. The low amounts of cholesterol and saturated fats will no add to plaque buildup in the arteries. And the plant-based diet is known to help relieve inflammation, which can also lead to heart disease. And since plants are rich in their levels of soluble fiber, they help to lower the levels of cholesterol in the body by slowing the body's absorption of cholesterol and reducing the amount the liver naturally produces.

Adult-onset diabetes or sugar diabetes are just alternative titles for Type 2 Diabetes. Type 1 Diabetes, the one most often diagnosed in childhood, is caused by the pancreas stopping the production of insulin. For some as yet unknown reasons, the pancreas ceases to function, and the body no longer produces insulin to carry the blood glucose into the cells. Type 2 Diabetes is generally preventable, and the reason it is often referred to as sugar diabetes is from the belief that people who consume too much sugar will get diabetes. This is partially true because a diet of highly processed foods that are high in sugar is one of the premier causes of Type 2 Diabetes.

When your body begins to resist the good effects of the insulin, it produces you begin metabolic syndrome. Your pancreas will make enough insulin and secrete it into your bloodstream to take the appropriate amount of glucose to your cells for energy. The problem starts when there is an excess of glucose in your bloodstream. When the cells are full, then the insulin will store the excess glucose as fat, and then the levels of glucose will drop back to normal. When this finely tuned production is thrown off course by excess food consumption, which causes excess insulin production, which causes excess glucose storage, then the levels of glucose will build up in your bloodstream, and this is when the diagnosis of diabetes happens. Being overweight is the single largest risk factor for the development of diabetes. Inactivity and abdominal fat are also risk factors.

A plant-based diet is crucial for reducing the risk of developing Type 2 Diabetes. For the best levels of health, the consumption of animal protein should be minimized. The plant-based diet can reduce the risk of developing Type 2 Diabetes by lowering the risk of gaining excessive amounts of weight. People who consume a plant-based diet typically eat less fat and fewer calories. They also consume less cholesterol and saturated fats while consuming more potassium and fiber, all of which will help to prevent or eliminate Type 2 Diabetes.

Cancer is a somewhat broad term that describes what happens when changes in the cells cause abnormal growth and division. Cancer will cause cells to divide uncontrollably, which will result in the formation of tumors and damage to your immune system. Most of the cells in your body have fixed lifespans and specific functions. Cells will naturally die during the course of your life, and new cells will take its place. Cancer cells know how to grow, but they lack the elements that tell them when to stop growing and when to die. They continue to grow in the body and use up nutrients and oxygen that the body could use in better ways. Some cancers are born with us and will appear at some time in our life, and those can't be prevented. But some cancers are caused by poor nutrition and the effects of excess body weight.

Being overweight is directly linked to the development of several types of cancers, including cancers of the pancreas, esophagus, kidney, rectum and colon, liver, and gallbladder. Excess body fat leads to inflammation and suppressed immune system function. It will hamper the production of certain hormones like estrogen and insulin. Being obese interferes with proper cell growth and production. And it can adversely affect the way in which the body uses certain hormones.

People who are obese usually have higher levels of inflammation, which can cause cell damage and are associated with digestive diseases that can lead to cancer of the rectum and colon. Also, people who are obese generally eat less fiber than is recommended. Fiber cleanses the colon and rectum as the waste product passes through and leaves less behind that can cause inflammations and diseases. Excess fat in your body can lead to the production of gall stones, which could lead to the development of cancer of the gallbladder.

Plant foods are excellent sources of substances that are called phytochemicals, and these can lead to protection from cancer-causing cells. The pigments that give bright colors to vegetables and fruits are the same substances that will help you prevent or fight cancer. And plant food contains fiber, which removes excess waste material and hormones from your body.

Replacing the animal protein in your diet with plant-based protein will lower your risk of death from heart disease and cancer. Plant-based proteins from foods such as grains, legumes, and vegetables can improve overall weight, cholesterol levels, and blood pressure. People who consume a plant-based diet have lower body mass indexes. They are more successful at keeping excess weight off. A plant-based diet will lower your risk of high blood pressure and cardiovascular disease. Your blood sugar levels and cholesterol levels will be easier to control. Your levels of inflammation will be reduced. Your risk of developing diabetes will be reduced. You will greatly benefit by lowering the amounts of animal substances you take in and increasing your consumption of beneficial plant-based foods.

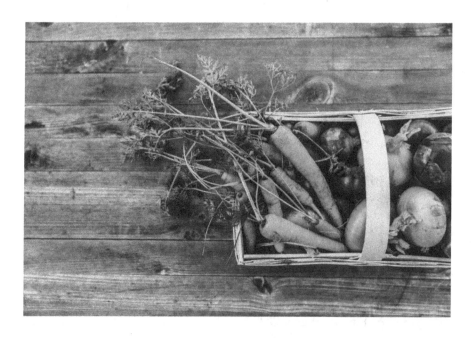

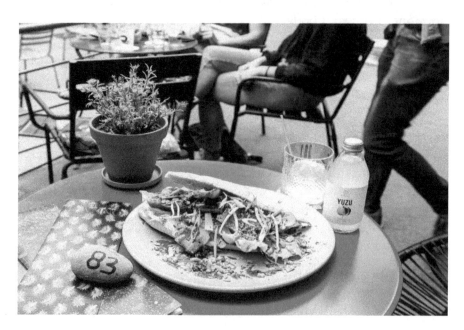

# Chapter 1.  Breakfasts

## 1.  Green Croquettes

Preparation time: 15 minutes

Cooking time: 5 minutes

Servings: 4

Ingredients:

2 sweet potatoes, peeled, boiled

1 cup fresh spinach

1 tablespoons peanuts

3 tablespoons flax meal

1 teaspoon salt

1 teaspoon ground black pepper

1 tablespoon olive oil

½ teaspoon dried oregano

¾ cup wheat flour

Directions:

Mash the sweet potatoes and place them in the mixing bowl. Add

flax meal salt, dried oregano, and ground black pepper.

Then blend the spinach with peanuts until smooth.

Add the green mixture in the sweet potato.

Mix up the mass.

Make medium size croquettes and coat them in the wheat flour.

Preheat instant pot on Saute mode well.

Add olive oil.

Roast croquettes for 1 minute from each side or until golden

brown.

Dry the cooked croquettes with a paper towel if needed.

Nutrition:

Calories 155, Total Fat 6.8g, Total Carbohydrate 20.6g, Protein 4.4g

## 2. Cigar Borek

Preparation time: 10 minutes

Cooking time: 5 minutes

Servings: 6

Ingredients:

6 oz phyllo dough

8 oz vegan Parmesan, grated

1 tablespoon vegan mayonnaise

1 teaspoon minced garlic

1 tablespoon avocado oil

Directions:

In the mixing bowl, mix up together grated Parmesan, vegan mayonnaise, and minced garlic.

Then cut phyllo dough into triangles.

Spread the triangles with cheese mixture and roll in the shape of cigars.

Preheat avocado oil in the instant pot on Saute mode.

Place rolled "cigar" in the instant pot and cook them for 1-2 minutes or until they are golden brown.

Nutrition:

Calories 210, Total Fat 2.6g, Total Carbohydrate 23.1g, Protein 17.5g

## 3. Flaked Clusters

Preparation time: 10 minutes

Cooking time: 4 minutes

Servings: 4

Ingredients:

3 oz chia seeds

½ cup pumpkin seeds

1 cup coconut flakes

1/3 cup maple syrup

1 cup water, for cooking

Directions:

In the mixing bowl mix up together chia seeds, pumpkin seeds, coconut flakes, and maple syrup.

Then line the trivet with the baking paper.

Pour water in the instant pot. Insert lined trivet.

With the help of 2 spoons make medium size clusters (patties) from the coconut mixture and put them on the trivet.

Close and seal the lid.

Cook clusters for 4 minutes on High.

Then use quick pressure release and open the lid.

Transfer the cooked clusters on the plate and let them chill well.

Nutrition:

Calories 336, Total Fat 21.2g, Total Carbohydrate 32.7g, Protein 8.4g

## 4. Marinara Sauce

Preparation time: 20 minutes

Cooking time: 20 minutes

Servings: 13

Ingredients:

4 28-oz. Cans diced tomatoes

1 cup fresh basil (chopped)

4 tbsp. Olive oil

4 tbsp. Nutritional yeast

6 medium garlic cloves (minced)

2 tsp. Dried oregano

1½ tbsp. Maple syrup

½ tsp. Cayenne pepper

Salt to taste

Directions:

Heat a large pot over medium heat.

Add the olive oil and minced garlic; sauté for about 1 minute.

Continue by adding the diced tomatoes, maple syrup, cayenne pepper, and oregano. Taste and add salt accordingly.

Bring the mixture to a simmer. Reduce the heat to low and cover the pot. Simmer the ingredients for about 25 minutes.

Add the basil and nutritional yeast. Stir well. Add more water if necessary.

Add more spices or salt to taste.

Incorporate the sauce in a dish, or store for future use.

Nutrition:

Calories 65, Total Fat 4.3g, Total Carbohydrate 4.9g, Protein 1.5g

## 5. Enchilada Sauce

Preparation time: 10 minutes

Cooking time: 10 minutes

Servings: 13

Ingredients:

1½ tbsp. Mct oil

½ tbsp. Chili powder

½ tbsp. Whole wheat flour

½ tsp. Ground cumin

¼ tsp. Oregano (dried or fresh)

¼ tsp. Salt (or to taste)

1 garlic clove (minced)

1 tbsp. Tomato paste

1 cup vegetable broth

½ tsp. Apple vinegar

½ tsp. Ground black pepper

Directions:

Heat a small saucepan over medium heat.

Add the mct oil and minced garlic to the pan and sauté for about 1 minute.

Mix the dry spices and flour in a medium bowl and pour the dry mixture into the sauce pan.

Stir in the tomato paste immediately, and slowly pour in the vegetable broth, making sure that everything combines well.

When everything is mixed thoroughly, bring up the heat to medium-high until it gets to a simmer and cook for about 3 minutes or until the sauce becomes a bit thicker.

Remove the pan from the heat and add the vinegar with the black pepper, adding more salt and pepper to taste.

Nutrition:

Calories 18, Total Fat 16g, Total Carbohydrate 0.6g, Protein 0.1g

## 6. Mexican Salsa

Preparation time: 10 minutes

Cooking time: 10 minutes

Servings: 6

Ingredients:

4 large, firm tomatoes

1 fresh jalapeno

½ medium red onion

2 tbsp. Fresh cilantro (chopped)

1 lime

Salt & black pepper to taste

Directions:

Skin and seed tomatoes.

Halve the jalapeno; remove and discard stem, seeds, and placenta.

Cut the tomatoes and jalapeno into fine pieces and add to bowl.

Finely chop the cilantro and red onion and add to bowl.

Juice the lime into the bowl.

Mix the ingredients and season to taste with salt and black pepper.

Let sit for 1 hour before serving.

Nutrition:

Calories 30, Total Fat 0.3g, Total Carbohydrate 6.1g, Protein 0.8g

## 7. Apple Sauce

Preparation time: 20 minutes

Cooking time: 20 minutes

Servings: 4

Ingredients:

4 jazz apples (peeled, cored, and quartered)

4 red delicious apples (peeled, cored, and quartered)

½ cup water

1 pinch salt

½ tsp. Cinnamon (optional)

1 tbsp. Lemon juice (optional)

Directions:

Put the apples into cold water for about 5 minutes.

Remove the apples from the water and further cut the quarters into

slices.

The Plant-Based Diet Mastery

Cook the slices of apple in a saucepan over medium heat with the water and salt.

Stir often and bring down to a simmer after it starts to cook.

After about 10 minutes of cooking, mash the apples while they are still simmering to create a sauce. Continue stirring and mashing further for about 20 minutes until you have a chunky apple sauce.

Add optional cinnamon and/or lemon juice if preferred.

Let it cool.

Nutrition:

Calories 202, Total Fat 9g, Total Carbohydrate 50g, Protein 8.4g

## 8.  Vegan Mayo

Preparation time: 10 minutes

Cooking time: 0 minutes

Servings: 6

Ingredients:

1 cup mct oil

1 tsp. Lemon juice

½ cup almond milk

1 tsp. Agave nectar

1 tsp. Rice vinegar

½ tsp. Mustard (ground)

1 tsp. Onion powder (optional)  1 tsp. Chili powder (optional)

1 tsp. Paprika powder (optional)   garlic clove (optional)

Directions:

Put the almond milk, agave nectar, rice vinegar, mustard, and if desired, the optional ingredients into a blender and blend.

Slowly add the mct oil to the blender while blending to emulsify the oil

and almond milk.

When the mixture starts to thicken, add the lemon juice.

Store in a sealable glass jar.

Nutrition:

Calories 344, Total Fat 37.5g, Total Carbohydrate 1.3g, Protein 1.5g

## 9. Chickpea Veggie Omelets

Preparation Time: 5 minutes

Cooking Time: 15 minutes

Servings: 1

Ingredients:

Water - .33 cup

Chickpea flour - .25 cup

Sea salt - .5 teaspoon

Nutritional yeast – 1 tablespoon

Bell pepper, red, diced – 2 tablespoons

Onion, diced – 2 tablespoons

Kale, chopped - .25 cup

Avocado oil – 1 tablespoon

Turmeric - .25 teaspoon

Garlic powder - .25 teaspoon

Black pepper, ground – dash

Directions:

In a small bowl whisk together the sea salt, nutritional yeast, chickpea flour, turmeric, garlic powder, ground black pepper, and water until it is completely smooth without any lumps remaining. Set the chickpea mixture aside while you prepare the vegetables.

Over a temperature of medium heat on the stove place a medium non-stick skillet with the avocado oil in the pan. Place the vegetables into the avocado oil and allow them to cook until tender, about five minutes.

Once you have cooked the onion, kale, and red bell pepper for five minutes, remove them from the non-stick skillet and add them to the chickpea mixture, whisking the ingredients completely together.

Pour the batter with the vegetables into the skillet, and cook it as if it were a pancake. You will know that the omelet is ready to flip once the top of the batter no longer appears wet to the eyes, about five minutes.

The Plant-Based Diet Mastery

Once your omelet has cooked for about five minutes, use a large spatula, and carefully flip it over, cooking the other side of the chickpea omelet for three to five minutes. You want to cook it until it is cooked through with no wet batter remaining in the center.

Flip half of the omelet over on top of itself so that it is in an omelet shape. You can serve it either as-is or sprinkle your favorite vegan cheese into the center before flipping the cooked omelet over onto itself.

Nutrition:

Number of Calories in Individual Servings: 254

Protein Grams: 8

Fat Grams: 15

Total Carbohydrates Grams: 20

Net Carbohydrates Grams: 16

## 10. Maple Cinnamon French Toast

Preparation Time: 5 minutes

Cooking Time: 15 minutes

Servings: 1

Ingredients:

Tofu, extra-firm – 4.5 ounces or .33 cup

Soy milk, unsweetened – 1 cup

Cinnamon, ground - .5 teaspoon

Maple syrup – 2 tablespoons

Sea salt - .25 teaspoon Vanilla extract – 2 teaspoons

White bread, thickly sliced and stale – 6 slices

Coconut oil – 1 tablespoon

Directions:

In a blender add in the tofu, soy milk, cinnamon, maple syrup, sea salt, and vanilla extract. You want to blend the tofu mixture until it is completely smooth with no lumps remaining.

Place a large non-stick skillet on the stove over med-low heat or set an electric griddle to the temperature of three-hundred and fifty degrees Fahrenheit.

Place the stale bread slices in a large bowl or a nine-by-thirteen baking dish and then pour the tofu mixture over the bread. You need to allow the bread to soak up the tofu mixture for about thirty seconds, flip the bread over, and allow it to soak up the mixture for an additional thirty seconds. If any area of the bread is still dry dip it into the tofu mixture to ensure it is evenly coated.

Pour the coconut oil into the non-stick skillet or griddle and use a pastry brush to ensure it is evenly coating the entire cooking surface. Place the soaked bread slices onto the pan, leaving enough room between slices to flip them over.

Cook the first side of the vegan French toast for four to five minutes before gently flipping them over and cooking for an additional four to five minutes. You want the color to be a light golden, be careful to not burn them! It is important to let the French toast cook without moving it around or messing with the slices. If you try to peek at the slices by moving them around, then it will damage the toast, possibly causing it to fall apart.

Once both sides of the toast are cooked, remove it from the pan and serve with your favorite toppings.

Nutrition:

Number of Calories in Individual Servings: 281

Protein Grams: 12

Fat Grams: 9

Total Carbohydrates Grams: 36

Net Carbohydrates Grams: 31

## 11. Savory Sweet Potato Oven Hash

Preparation Time: 10 minutes Cooking Time: 60 minutes

Servings: 6

Ingredients:

Sweet potatoes, peeled, diced into one-inch cubes – 6 cups, about 2-3

large potatoes

Onion, diced – 1 medium Onion powder – 1 teaspoon

Olive oil - .25 cup Sea salt – 2 teaspoons

Thyme, dried – 1 teaspoon Paprika - .5 teaspoon

Garlic powder – 1 tablespoon Garlic, minced – 12 cloves

Directions:

While the oven preheats to a temperature of four-hundred and fifty

degrees prepare the sweet potatoes, onion, and garlic. Be sure to wash

the sweet potatoes and cut them with a sharp knife to prevent

accidents. Using a dull knife will cause the knife to slip and increase

the risk of injuries, using a large sharp knife is much safer.

Place the diced sweet potatoes into a large nine-by-thirteen glass pan along with the seasonings and the olive oil, tossing the ingredients together completely. Allow the sweet potatoes to cook in the preheated oven for forty-five minutes, stirring them every fifteen minutes to allow for even cooking and to prevent burning.

After the forty-five minutes are up add in the diced onion and minced garlic, tossing the ingredients together. Allow the mixture to cook for an additional fifteen minutes until the onions and garlic are caramelized.

Remove the hash from the oven, give it one good last stir to combine, and serve! You can either enjoy this hash alone or with your favorite tofu scramble or vegan breakfast sausage.

Nutrition:Number of Calories in Individual Servings: 218

Protein Grams: 3 Fat Grams: 9 Total Carbohydrates Grams: 32

Net Carbohydrates Grams: 28

## 12. Lemon Poppy Seed Pancakes

Preparation Time: 5 minutes Cooking Time: 15 minutes

Servings: 3

Ingredients:

White whole-wheat flour – 1 cup Poppy seeds – 1 tablespoon

Sea salt - .5 teaspoon Bob's Red Mill Egg Replacer – 1 tablespoon

Water – 2 tablespoons Baking Soda – 1 tablespoon

Oat milk – .75 cup Lemon zest – 1 tablespoon

Lemon juice - .25 cup

Sugar – 2 tablespoons

Coconut oil – 1 tablespoon

Directions:

Combine the oat milk and lemon juice in a measuring cup and allow it

to sit for five minutes. This will help make the oat milk into faux

buttermilk. Once it has set stir in the lemon zest and sugar. Set the oat

milk mixture aside.

In a large bowl whisk together the white whole-wheat flour, baking soda, sea salt, and chia seeds. Set the wheat flour mixture aside.

In a small serving bowl whisk together the Egg Replacer and water until it is free of clumps and thickens. Pour the thickened egg mixture into the oat milk mixture.

Once the wet ingredients are all combined, add them into the whole-wheat flour mixture and stir until just combined. You want to stir until the lumps are removed, but you don't want to over mix the batter. When pancake batter is overmixed, it will cause the baking soda to lose its effectiveness, therefore making the pancakes less fluffy.

While the prepared pancake batter rests, allow a large non-stick skillet to heat over medium heat or an electric griddle to heat over three-hundred- and sixty-degrees Fahrenheit.

Once your electric griddle or non-stick skillet are preheated use a pastry brush to coat the surface with the coconut oil. Use a scoop to measure out the pancake batter into rounds on the cooking surface, with each pancake being between .25-.5 cups of batter. Ensure that each pancake has enough space between them so that you can easily flip the pancakes once cooked.

You will know the pancakes are ready to flip once they begin to look dry around the edges and the bubbles that form in the center pop. Flip the pancakes once they reach this stage, which should take three to five minutes. Cook the other side of the pancakes for two to three minutes until golden brown.

Remove the pancakes from the cooking surface and serve with your favorite toppings.

Nutrition:

Number of Calories in Individual Servings: 311

Protein Grams: 6

Fat Grams: 12

Total Carbohydrates Grams: 50 Net Carbohydrates Grams: 44

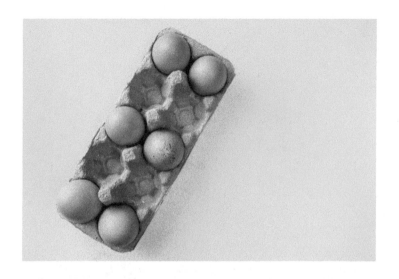

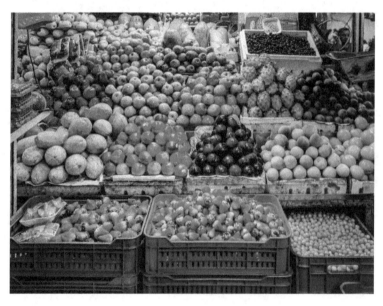

# Chapter 2.  : Salads, Soups, and Sides

## 13. Zucchini Soup

Preparation Time: 20 minutes

Cooking Time: 20 minutes

Servings: 8

Ingredients:

2 ½ lbs zucchini, peeled and sliced

1/3 cup basil leaves

4 cups vegetable stock

4 garlic cloves, chopped

2 tbsp olive oil

1 medium onion, diced

Pepper

Salt

Directions:

Heat olive oil in a pan over medium-low heat.

Add zucchini and onion and sauté until softened. Add garlic and sauté

for a minute.

Add vegetable stock and simmer for 15 minutes.

Remove from heat. Stir in basil and puree the soup using a blender

until smooth and creamy. Season with pepper and salt.

Stir well and serve.

Nutrition:

Calories 62

Fat 4 g

Carbohydrates 6.8 g

Sugar 3.3 g

Protein 2 g

Cholesterol 0 mg

## 14. Creamy Celery Soup

Preparation Time: 40 minutes

Cooking Time: 10 minutes

Servings: 4

Ingredients:

6 cups celery

½ tsp dill

2 cups water

1 cup coconut milk

1 onion, chopped

Pinch of salt

Directions:

Add all ingredients into the electric pot and stir well.

Cover electric pot with the lid and select soup setting.

Release pressure using a quick release method than open the lid.

Puree the soup using an immersion blender until smooth and creamy.

Stir well and serve warm.

Nutrition:

Calories 174

Fat 14.6 g

Carbohydrates 10.5 g

Sugar 5.2 g

Protein 2.8 g

Cholesterol 0 mg

## 15. Avocado Cucumber Soup

Preparation Time: 40 minutes

Cooking Time: 0 minutes

Servings:

Ingredients:

1 large cucumber, peeled and sliced

¾ cup water

¼ cup lemon juice

2 garlic cloves

6 green onion

2 avocados, pitted

½ tsp black pepper

½ tsp pink salt

Directions:

Add all ingredients into the blender and blend until smooth and

creamy.

Place in refrigerator for 30 minutes.

Stir well and serve chilled.

Nutrition:

Calories 73

Fat 3.7 g

Carbohydrates 9.2 g

Sugar 2.8 g

Protein 2.2 g

Cholesterol 0 mg

## 16. Creamy Garlic Onion Soup

Preparation Time: 45 minutes

Cooking Time: 25 minutes

Servings: 4

Ingredients:

1 onion, sliced

4 cups vegetable stock

1 1/2 tbsp olive oil

1 shallot, sliced

2 garlic clove, chopped

1 leek, sliced

Salt

Directions:

Add stock and olive oil in a saucepan and bring to boil.

Add remaining ingredients and stir well.

Cover and simmer for 25 minutes.

Puree the soup using an immersion blender until smooth.

Stir well and serve warm.

Nutrition:

Calories 90

Fat 7.4 g

Carbohydrates 10.1g

Sugar 4.1 g

Protein 1 g

Cholesterol 0 mg

## 17. Avocado Broccoli Soup

Preparation Time: 25 minutes  Cooking Time: 5 minutes

Servings: 4

Ingredients:

2 cups broccoli florets, chopped  5 cups vegetable broth

2 avocados, chopped  Pepper

Salt

Directions:

Cook broccoli in boiling water for 5 minutes. Drain well.

Add broccoli, vegetable broth, avocados, pepper, and salt to the

blender and blend until smooth.  Stir well and serve warm.

Nutrition:

Calories 269 Fat 21.5 g Carbohydrates 12.8 g Sugar 2.1 g

Protein 9.2 g

Cholesterol 0 mg

# Chapter 3. : Entrées

## 18. Super tasty Vegetarian Chili

Preparation Time: 20 minutes

Cooking Time: 2 hours and 10 minutes

Servings: 6

Ingredients:

16-ounce of vegetarian baked beans

16 ounce of cooked chickpeas

16 ounce of cooked kidney beans

15 ounce of cooked corn

1 medium-sized green bell pepper, cored and chopped

2 stalks of celery, peeled and chopped

12 ounce of chopped tomatoes

1 medium-sized white onion, peeled and chopped

1 teaspoon of minced garlic  1 teaspoon of salt

1 tablespoon of red chili powder  1 tablespoon of dried oregano

1 tablespoon of dried basil  1 tablespoon of dried parsley

18-ounce of black bean soup  4-ounce of tomato puree

Directions:

Take a 6-quarts slow cooker, grease it with a non-stick cooking spray and place all the ingredients into it.

Stir properly and cover the top.

Plug in the slow cooker; adjust the cooking time to 2 hours and let it cook on the high heat setting or until it is cooked thoroughly.

Serve right away.

Nutrition:

Calories: 190 Cal arbohydrates: 35g

Protein: 11g Fats: 1g Fiber: 10g

## 19. Creamy Sweet Potato & Coconut Curry

Preparation Time: 15 minutes

Cooking Time: 6 hours and 20 minutes

Servings: 6

Ingredients:

2 pounds of sweet potatoes, peeled and chopped

1/2 pound of red cabbage, shredded

2 red chilies, seeded and sliced

2 medium-sized red bell peppers, cored and sliced

2 large white onions, peeled and sliced

1 1/2 teaspoon of minced garlic

1 teaspoon of grated ginger

1/2 teaspoon of salt

1 teaspoon of paprika

1/2 teaspoon of cayenne pepper

2 tablespoons of peanut butter

4 tablespoons of olive oil

12-ounce of tomato puree

14 fluid ounce of coconut milk

1/2 cup of chopped coriander

Directions:

Place a large non-stick skillet pan over an average heat, add 1 tablespoon of oil and let it heat.

Then add the onion and cook for 10 minutes or until it gets soft.

Add the garlic, ginger, salt, paprika, cayenne pepper and continue cooking for 2 minutes or until it starts producing fragrance.

Transfer this mixture to a 6-quarts slow cooker and reserve the pan.

In the pan, add 1 tablespoon of oil and let it heat.

Add the cabbage, red chili, bell pepper and cook it for 5 minutes.

Then transfer this mixture to the slow cooker and reserve the pan.

Add the remaining oil to the pan; the sweet potatoes in a single layer and cook it in 3 batches for 5 minutes or until it starts getting brown.

Add the sweet potatoes to the slow cooker, along with tomato puree, coconut milk and stir properly.

Cover the top, plug in the slow cooker; adjust the cooking time to 6 hours and let it cook on the low heat setting or until the sweet potatoes are tender.

When done, add the seasoning and pour it in the peanut butter.

Garnish it with coriander and serve.

Nutrition:

Calories: 434 Cal

Carbohydrates: 47g

Protein: 6g

Fats: 22g

Fiber: 3g.

## 20. Comforting Chickpea Tagine

Preparation Time: 20 minutes

Cooking Time: 4 hours and 15 minutes

Servings: 6

Ingredients:

14 ounce of cooked chickpeas

12 dried apricots

1 red bell pepper, cored and sliced

1 small butternut squash, peeled, cored and chopped

2 zucchini, stemmed and chopped

1 medium-sized white onion, peeled and chopped

1 teaspoon of minced garlic

1 teaspoon of ground ginger

1 1/2 teaspoon of salt

1 teaspoon of ground black pepper

1 teaspoon of ground cumin

2 teaspoon of paprika

1 teaspoon of harissa paste

2 teaspoon of honey

2 tablespoons of olive oil

1 pound of passata

1/4 cup of chopped coriander

Directions:

Take a 6-quarts slow cooker, grease it with a non-stick cooking spray and place the chickpeas, apricots, bell pepper, butternut squash, zucchini and onion into it.

Sprinkle it with salt, black pepper and set it aside until it is called for.

Place a large non-stick skillet pan over an average temperature of heat; add the oil, garlic, cumin and paprika.

Stir properly and cook for 1 minutes or until it starts producing fragrance.

Then pour in the harissa paste, honey, passata and boil the mixture.

When the mixture is done boiling, pour this mixture over the vegetables in the slow cooker and cover it with the lid.

Plug in the slow cooker; adjust the cooking time to 4 hours and let it cook on the high heat setting or until the vegetables gets tender.

When done, add the seasoning, garnish it with the coriander and serve right away.

Nutrition:

Calories: 237 Cal

Carbohydrates: 45g

Protein: 9g

Fats: 2g

Fiber: 8g.

## 21. Brown Basmati Rice Pilaf

Preparation Time: 10 minutes

Cooking Time: 3 minutes

Servings: 2

Ingredients:

½ tablespoon vegan butter

½ cup mushrooms, chopped

½ cup brown basmati rice

2-3 tablespoons water

1/8 teaspoon dried thyme

Ground pepper to taste

½ tablespoon olive oil

¼ cup green onion, chopped

1 cup vegetable broth

¼ teaspoon salt

¼ cup chopped, toasted pecans

Directions:

Place a saucepan over medium-low heat. Add butter and oil.

When it melts, add mushrooms and cook until slightly tender.

Stir in the green onion and brown rice. Cook for 3 minutes. Stir

constantly.

Stir in the broth, water, salt and thyme.

When it begins to boil, lower heat and cover with a lid. Simmer until

rice is cooked. Add more water or broth if required.

Stir in the pecans and pepper.

Serve.

Nutrition:

Calories 189

Fats 11 g

Carbohydrates 19 g

Proteins 4 g

## 22. Mexican Rice

Preparation Time: 10 minutes

Cooking Time: 15 minutes

Servings: 4

Ingredients:

½ can diced tomatoes with its liquid

2 ounces corn

½ can tomatoes with green chilies with its liquid

1 small onion, chopped

½ can black beans, drained, rinsed

1 small green bell pepper, chopped

1 tablespoon olive oil

½ cup white rice

¾ cup water

2 -3 tablespoons picante style salsa

2 tablespoons black olives, pitted, sliced

1 jalapeno pepper, sliced

Vegan sour cream to serve

Vegan cheese, shredded to serve

Directions:

Place a pan over medium heat. Add oil. When the oil is heated, add bell pepper and onions and sauté until tender.

Add rest of the ingredients except vegan sour cream and cheese. Stir and bring to the boil.

Lower the heat. Cover and cook for 15 minutes until rice is tender.

Serve garnished with vegan sour cream and cheese.

Nutrition:

Calories 133.8

Fats 0.7 g

Carbohydrates 27.5 g

Proteins 6.1 g

## 23. Artichoke & Eggplant Rice

Preparation Time: 5 minutes

Cooking Time: 10 minutes

Servings: 3

Ingredients:

2 tablespoons olive oil

1 medium onion, finely chopped

A handful parsley, chopped

1 teaspoon turmeric powder

3 cups vegetable stock

Juice, lemon

1 eggplant, chopped into chunks

1 clove garlic, crushed

1 teaspoon smoked paprika

7 ounces paella rice

1 package chargrilled artichoke

Lemon wedges to serve

Directions:

Place a nonstick pan or paella pan over medium heat. Add 1 tablespoon oil. When the oil is heated, add eggplant and cook until brown all over.

Remove with a slotted spoon and place on a plate lined with paper towels.

Add 1 tablespoon oil. When the oil is heated, add onion and sauté until translucent.

Stir in garlic and parsley stalks. Cook for 10 minutes. Add all the spices and rice and stir-fry for a few minutes until rice is well coated with the oil.

Add salt and mix well. Pour half the broth and cook until dry. Stir occasionally.

Add eggplant and artichokes and stir. Pour remaining stock and cook until rice is tender. Add parsley leaves and lemon juice and stir.

Serve hot with lemon wedges.

Nutrition:

Calories 431

Fats 16 g

Carbohydrates 58 g

Proteins 8 g

## 24. Black Beans and Rice

Preparation Time: 6 minutes

Cooking Time: 15 minutes

Servings: 3

Ingredients:

1 tablespoon vegetable oil

½ can

1 ½ teaspoons dried oregano

½ cup uncooked rice

1 large onion, chopped

¼ teaspoon creole seasoning

¼ teaspoon ground cumin

¾ teaspoon garlic powder

½ teaspoon salt or to taste

1 cup water

Cilantro to garnish

Directions:

Place a saucepan over medium heat. Add oil. When the oil is heated, add onions and sauté until tender. Add rest of the ingredients except rice and beans and mix well.

When it begins to boil, add rice and mix well.

Lower the heat and cover with a lid. Simmer for 15 minutes until rice is tender.

Turn off the heat. Let it sit covered for 5 minutes.

Fluff with a fork. Add beans and stir. Cover and let it sit for 5 minutes.

Garnish with cilantro if desired and serve.

Nutrition:

Calories 233

Fats 5 g

Carbohydrates 39.9 g

Proteins 7 g

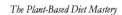

# Chapter 4. : Smoothies and

# Beverages

### 25. Spiced Strawberry Smoothie

Preparation Time: 5 minutes

Cooking Time: 0 minute

Servings: 1

Ingredients:

1 tablespoon goji berries, soaked

1 cup strawberries

1/8 teaspoon sea salt

1 frozen banana

1 Medjool date, pitted

1 scoop vanilla-flavored whey protein

2 tablespoons lemon juice

¼ teaspoon ground ginger

½ teaspoon ground cinnamon

1 tablespoon almond butter

1 cup almond milk, unsweetened

Directions:

Place all the ingredients in the order in a food processor or blender

and then pulse for 2 to 3 minutes at high speed until smooth.

Pour the smoothie into a glass and then serve.

Nutrition:

Calories: 182 Cal

Fat: 1.3 g

Carbs: 34 g

Protein: 6.4 g

Fiber: 0.7 g

## 26. Banana Bread Shake With Walnut Milk

Preparation Time: 5 minutes    Cooking Time: 0 minute

Servings: 2

Ingredients:

2 cups sliced frozen bananas  3 cups walnut milk

1/8 teaspoon grated nutmeg  1 tablespoon maple syrup

1 teaspoon ground cinnamon

1/2 teaspoon vanilla extract, unsweetened  2 tablespoons cacao nibs

Directions:

Place all the ingredients in the order in a food processor or blender and then pulse for 2 to 3 minutes at high speed until smooth.

Pour the smoothie into two glasses and then serve.

Nutrition:

Calories: 339.8 Cal  Fat: 19 g  Carbs: 39 g

Protein: 4.3 g

## 27. Double Chocolate Hazelnut Espresso Shake

Preparation Time: 5 minutes

Cooking Time: 0 minute

Servings: 1

Ingredients:

1 frozen banana, sliced

1/4 cup roasted hazelnuts

4 Medjool dates, pitted, soaked

2 tablespoons cacao nibs, unsweetened

1 1/2 tablespoons cacao powder, unsweetened

1/8 teaspoon sea salt  1 teaspoon vanilla extract, unsweetened

1 cup almond milk, unsweetened

1/2 cup ice  4 ounces espresso, chilled

Directions:

Place all the ingredients in the order in a food processor or blender

and then pulse for 2 to 3 minutes at high speed until smooth.

Pour the smoothie into a glass and then serve.

Nutrition:

Calories: 210 Cal

Fat: 5 g

Carbs: 27 g

Protein: 16.8 g

Fiber: 0.2 g

## 28. Strawberry, Banana and Coconut Shake

Preparation Time: 5 minutes  Cooking Time: 0 minute

Servings: 1

Ingredients:

1 tablespoon coconut flakes  1 1/2 cups frozen banana slices

8 strawberries, sliced  1/2 cup coconut milk, unsweetened

1/4 cup strawberries for topping

Directions:

Place all the ingredients in the order in a food processor or blender, except for topping and then pulse for 2 to 3 minutes at high speed until smooth.

Pour the smoothie into a glass and then serve.

Nutrition:

Calories: 335 Cal  Fat: 5 g  Carbs: 75 g  Protein: 4 g

Fiber: 9 g

## 29. Tropical Vibes Green Smoothie

Preparation Time: 5 minutes

Cooking Time: 0 minute

Servings: 1

Ingredients:

2 stalks of kale, ripped

1 frozen banana

1 mango, peeled, pitted, chopped

1/8 teaspoon sea salt

¼ cup of coconut yogurt

½ teaspoon vanilla extract, unsweetened

1 tablespoon ginger juice

½ cup of orange juice  ½ cup of coconut water

Directions:

Place all the ingredients in the order in a food processor or blender

and then pulse for 2 to 3 minutes at high speed until smooth.

Pour the smoothie into a glass and then serve.

Nutrition:

Calories: 197.5 Cal

Fat: 1.3 g

Carbs: 30 g

Protein: 16.3 g

Fiber: 4.8 g

# Chapter 5. : Snacks and Desserts

---

### 30. Vegan Fudge Revel Bars

Preparation Time: 1 hour

Cooking Time: 0 minutes

Servings: 12

Ingredients:

1 cup almond flour

¾ cup erythritol

¾ cup peanut butter   1 tbsp vanilla extract

½ cup sugar-free chocolate chips

2 tbsp margarine

Directions:

Mix together almond butter, coconut flour, erythritol, and vanilla extract in a bowl until well combined.

The Plant-Based Diet Mastery

Press the mixture into a rectangular silicone mold and freeze for an

hour to set.

Melt the chocolate chips with the margarine for 1-2 minutes in the

microwave.

Pour melted chocolate on top of the mold and chill for another hour

to set.

Slice for serving.

Nutrition:

Calories 160

Carbohydrates 5 g

Fats 14 g

Protein 5 g

## 31. Nori Snack Rolls

Preparation Time: 5 minutes

Cooking Time: 10 minutes

Servings: 4 rolls

Ingredients:

2 tablespoons almond, cashew, peanut, or others nut butter

2 tablespoons tamari, or soy sauce

4 standard nori sheets

1 mushroom, sliced

1 tablespoon pickled ginger

½ cup grated carrots

Directions:

Preparing the Ingredients.

Preheat the oven to 350°F.

Mix together the nut butter and tamari until smooth and very thick.

Lay out a nori sheet, rough side up, the long way.

Spread a thin line of the tamari mixture on the far end of the nori sheet, from side to side. Lay the mushroom slices, ginger, and carrots in a line at the other end (the end closest to you).

Fold the vegetables inside the nori, rolling toward the tahini mixture, which will seal the roll. Repeat to make 4 rolls.

Put on a baking sheet and bake for 8 to 10 minutes, or until the rolls are slightly browned and crispy at the ends. Let the rolls cool for a few minutes, then slice each roll into 3 smaller pieces.

Nutrition:

Calories: 79

Total Fat: 5g

Carbs: 6g

Fiber: 2g

Protein: 4g

## 32. Risotto Bites

Preparation Time: 15 minutes

Cooking Time: 20 minutes

Servings: 12 bites

Ingredients:

½ cup panko bread crumbs

1 teaspoon paprika

1 teaspoon chipotle powder or ground cayenne pepper

1½ cups cold Green Pea Risotto

Nonstick cooking spray

Directions:

Preparing the Ingredients.

Preheat the oven to 425°F.

Line a baking sheet with parchment paper.

On a large plate, combine the panko, paprika, and chipotle powder.

Set aside.

Roll 2 tablespoons of the risotto into a ball.

Gently roll in the bread crumbs, and place on the prepared baking sheet. Repeat to make a total of 12 balls.

Spritz the tops of the risotto bites with nonstick cooking spray and bake for 15 to 20 minutes, until they begin to brown. Cool completely before storing in a large airtight container in a single layer (add a piece of parchment paper for a second layer) or in a plastic freezer bag.

Nutrition:

Calories: 100

Fat: 2g

Protein: 6g

Carbohydrates: 17g

Fiber: 5g

Sugar: 2g

Sodium: 165 mg

## 33. Tamari Toasted Almonds

Preparation Time: 2 minutes

Cooking Time: 8 minutes

Servings: ½ cup

Ingredients:

½ cup raw almonds, or sunflower seeds

2 tablespoons tamari, or soy sauce

1 teaspoon toasted sesame oil

Directions:

Preparing the Ingredients.

Heat a dry skillet to medium-high heat, then add the almonds, stirring very frequently to keep them from burning. Once the almonds are toasted, 7 to 8 minutes for almonds, or 3 to 4 minutes for sunflower seeds, pour the tamari and sesame oil into the hot skillet and stir to coat.

You can turn off the heat, and as the almonds cool the tamari mixture

will stick to and dry on the nuts.

Nutrition:

Calories: 89

Total Fat: 8g

Carbs: 3g

Fiber: 2g

Protein: 4g

## 34. Kale Chips

Preparation Time: 5 minutes

Cooking Time: 25 minutes

Servings: 2

Ingredients:

1 large bunch kale

1 tablespoon extra-virgin olive oil

½ teaspoon chipotle powder

½ teaspoon smoked paprika

¼ teaspoon salt

Directions:

Preparing the Ingredients.

Preheat the oven to 275°F.

Line a large baking sheet with parchment paper. In a large bowl, stem the kale and tear it into bite-size pieces. Add the olive oil, chipotle powder, smoked paprika, and salt.

Toss the kale with tongs or your hands, coating each piece well.

Spread the kale over the parchment paper in a single layer.

Bake for 25 minutes, turning halfway through, until crisp.

Cool for 10 to 15 minutes before dividing and storing in 2 airtight containers.

Nutrition: 144

Fat: 7g

Protein: 5g

Carbohydrates: 18g

Fiber: 3g

Sugar: 0g

Sodium: 363mg

## 35. Savory Seed Crackers

Preparation Time: 5 minutes

Cooking Time: 50 minutes

Servings: 20 crackers

Ingredients:

¾ cup pumpkin seeds (pepitas)

½ cup sunflower seeds

½ cup sesame seeds

¼ cup chia seeds

1 teaspoon minced garlic (about 1 clove)

1 teaspoon tamari or soy sauce

1 teaspoon vegan Worcestershire sauce

½ teaspoon ground cayenne pepper

½ teaspoon dried oregano ½ cup water

Directions:

Preparing the Ingredients.

Preheat the oven to 325°F.

Line a rimmed baking sheet with parchment paper.

In a large bowl, combine the pumpkin seeds, sunflower seeds, sesame seeds, chia seeds, garlic, tamari, Worcestershire sauce, cayenne, oregano, and water.

Transfer to the prepared baking sheet, spreading out to all sides.

Bake for 25 minutes. Remove the pan from the oven and flip the seed "dough" over so the wet side is up. Bake for another 20 to 25 minutes, until the sides are browned.

Cool completely before breaking up into 20 pieces. Divide evenly among 4 glass jars and close tightly with lids.

Nutrition:

Calories: 339 Fat: 29g Protein: 14g

Carbohydrates: 17g Fiber: 8g Sugar: 1g

Sodium: 96mg

## 36. Mushroom Bites

Preparation Time: 10 minutes

Cooking Time: 20 minutes

Servings: 4

Ingredients:

1 pound baby Bella mushroom caps

1 teaspoon garlic powder

2 tablespoons olive oil

Salt and black pepper to the taste

1 teaspoon curry powder

1 tablespoon parsley, chopped

Directions:

In a bowl, mix the mushrooms with the oil, garlic powder and the other ingredients and toss well.

Spread the mushrooms on a baking sheet lined with parchment paper and cook in the oven at 350 degrees F for 20 minutes.

Arrange on a platter and serve as an appetizer.

Nutrition:

Calories 144

Fat 20

Fiber 3

Carbs 7

# Chapter 6.  : Sauces, Dressings, and

# Dips

## 37. Raspberry Sauce

Preparation Time: 15 minutes

Cooking Time: 10 minutes

Servings: 8

Ingredients:

¼ cup white sugar

2 cups fresh raspberries

2 tablespoons cornstarch

2 tablespoons fresh orange juice

¼ cup white sugar

1 cup cold water

Directions:

Put water and cornstarch in a bowl and beat well.

Add the cornstarch mixture and rest of the ingredients to a pan and cook over medium-low heat for about 5 minutes.

Let the ingredients simmer for about 5 more minutes to have a thick consistency.

Remove from the heat and cool to serve.

Nutrition:

Calories: 49

Net Carbs: 8.2gFat: 0.2g

Carbohydrates: 12.2gFiber: 2g

Sugar: 7.9gProtein: 0.4g

Sodium: 1mg

## 38. Baba Ganoush

Preparation Time: 15 minutes

Cooking Time: 20 minutes

Ingredients:

1 garlic clove, chopped

¼ teaspoon salt

2 tablespoons tahini

¼ cup fresh parsley, chopped

1 large eggplant, pricked with a fork

2 tablespoons fresh lemon juice

Directions:

Preheat the oven to 450 degrees F and line a baking sheet with foil

paper.

Place the eggplant on the baking sheet and roast for about 20 minutes.

Remove from the oven and allow to cool.

Scoop out the pulp after cutting the eggplant.

Put this pulp to a food processor along rest of the ingredients.

Dish out in a bowl and serve warm.

Nutrition:

Calories: 78

Net Carbs: 2.1gFat: 4.3g

Carbohydrates: 9gFiber: 4.9g

Sugar: 3.7gProtein: 2.6g

Sodium: 162g

## 39. Basil Pesto

Preparation Time: 15 minutes

Cooking Time: 0 minutes

Servings: 8

Ingredients:

3 tablespoons nutritional yeast

2 cups tightly packed fresh basil

1 tablespoon fresh lemon juice

2 garlic cloves, chopped roughly

½ cup extra-virgin olive oil

½ cup walnuts

Pinch of salt and ground black pepper

Directions:

Grind the basil, garlic, and walnuts in a food processor

Add olive oil to it while the motor is running and combine well.

Add the nutritional yeast, lemon juice, salt and black pepper to it.

Mix well and dish out to serve and enjoy.

Nutrition:

Calories: 173

Net Carbs: 0gFat: 17.5g

Carbohydrates: 2.9gFiber: 1.6g

Sugar: 0.2gProtein: 3.9g

Sodium: 3mg

## 40. Poppy Seed Dressing

Preparation Time: 15 minutes

Cooking Time: 0 minutes

Servings: 12

Ingredients:

2/3 cup unsweetened cashew milk

½ teaspoon red palm oil

½ cup fresh lemon juice

¼ cup maple syrup

¾ teaspoon salt

½ teaspoon Dijon mustard

1 cup raw cashews

1 tablespoon poppy seeds

Directions:

Put the cashews in a spice grinder and pulse until smooth.

Put the cashew milk, lemon juice, maple syrup, mustard, palm oil and salt along with ground cashews in a blender.

Pulse until smooth and dish out in a container.

Stir in the poppy seeds and refrigerate to chill for about 2 hours.

Drizzle over your favorite salad and serve to enjoy.

Nutrition:

Calories: 92

Net Carbs: 6.1gFat: 6g

Carbohydrates: 8.6gFiber: 0.5g

Sugar: 4.8gProtein: 2g

Sodium: 163mg

## 41. Cranberry Dressing

Preparation Time: 15 minutes

Cooking Time: 0 minutes

Servings: 18

Ingredients:

¼ cup rice vinegar

¼ cup Dijon mustard

¼ cup cranberry sauc

¼ cup apple cider vinegar

¼ cup walnut oil

1 cup vegetable oil

1 garlic clove, chopped

Salt and ground black pepper, as require

Directions:

Put rice vinegar, Dijon mustard, cranberry sauce, apple cider vinegar,

garlic, salt and black pepper in a blender and pulse until smooth.

Add walnut oil and vegetable and pulse to form a creamy mixture.

Dish out in a bowl and serve to enjoy.

Nutrition:

Calories: 124

Net Carbs: 0gFat: 13.3g

Carbohydrates: 0.6gFiber: 0.3g

Sugar: 0.1gProtein: 0.6g

Sodium: 40mg

# Conclusion

Plants are a good source of all nutrients and minerals. They have low cholesterol, good lipids, and anti-oxidant characteristics which help to detoxify the body from pollutants. A plant-based diet has a significant impact on health, skin, and the environment. Plant-based diet improves and provides shine to the skin. I have observed my clear skin with a glow after the adoption of plant-based food in the first month. This book is a complete guide for beginners who intend to reduce weight, strengthen muscles and bones, and health-related problems such as heart diseases, obesity, and metabolic syndromes.

Enjoy this book with all vegan recipes which will help you to decide your daily food.